# IT'S ALWAYS PERSONAL

Writers Kornered Publishing
The Healing Woman023 LLC
Text Copyright ©2021 Martina Lanier
Illustrations Copyright ©2021
All rights reserved.

ISBN: 978-1-7372257-9-9

No part of this book shall be used or reproduced in any manner whatsoever without written consent/permission except in the case of brief quotations embodied in critical articles and reviews. For more information address Writers Kornered Publishing

Books can be purchased in bulk by emailing writerskornered@gmail.com

First Edition; Special Edition

⭐ Hi, brave boys and girls! ⭐

My name is Reign the Star!

My friends Tai the Teddy, Addie the Caddy, and I have some important things we would like to speak with you about! ⭐ ⭐

We need you to listen very closely and pay attention.

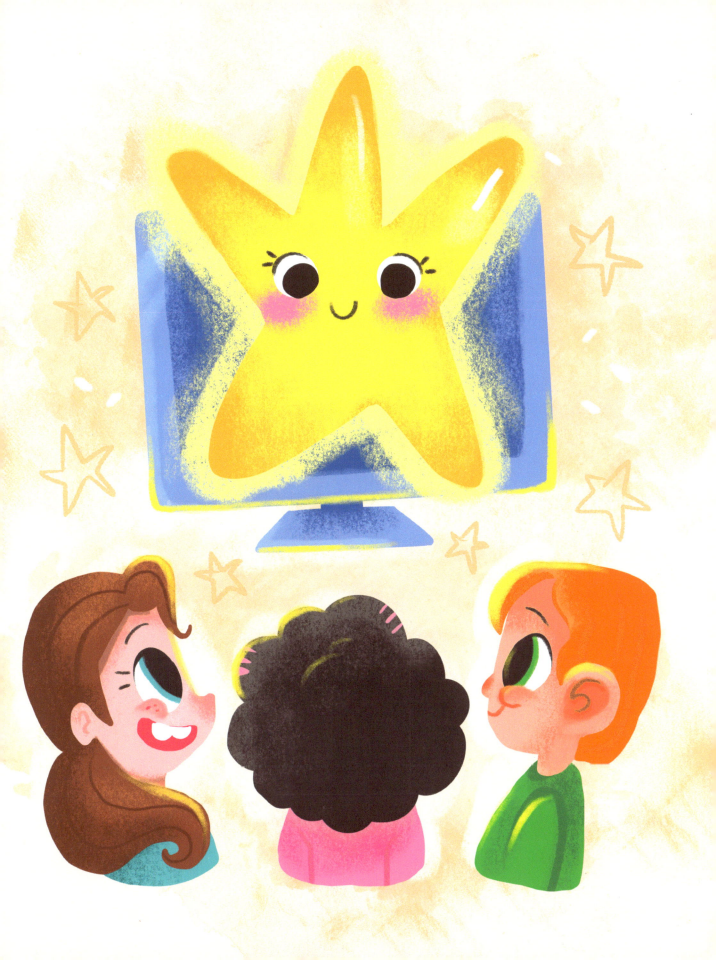

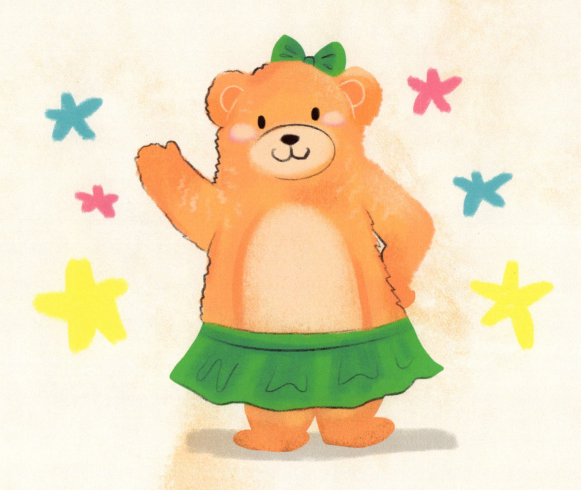

Hi! I'm Tai the Teddy, and I want to talk to you all about personal property and saying "No!"

YOU are your personal property—your head, arms, legs, and body are all personal, and they belong to YOU!

NO ONE should touch your personal property without your permission, and no one should ask YOU to touch other people's personal property, either.

Here—take a look at my picture. I put x's on all the parts of our bodies. Another person must have YOUR PERMISSION to touch any of these parts. I also put blank lines there, so you and your parents can talk about those body part names.

Now that you have the names of our very important and private body parts, let's talk about what we should do next.

If someone touches you and it makes you sad, mad, or uncomfortable, you should always tell someone— QUICKLY!

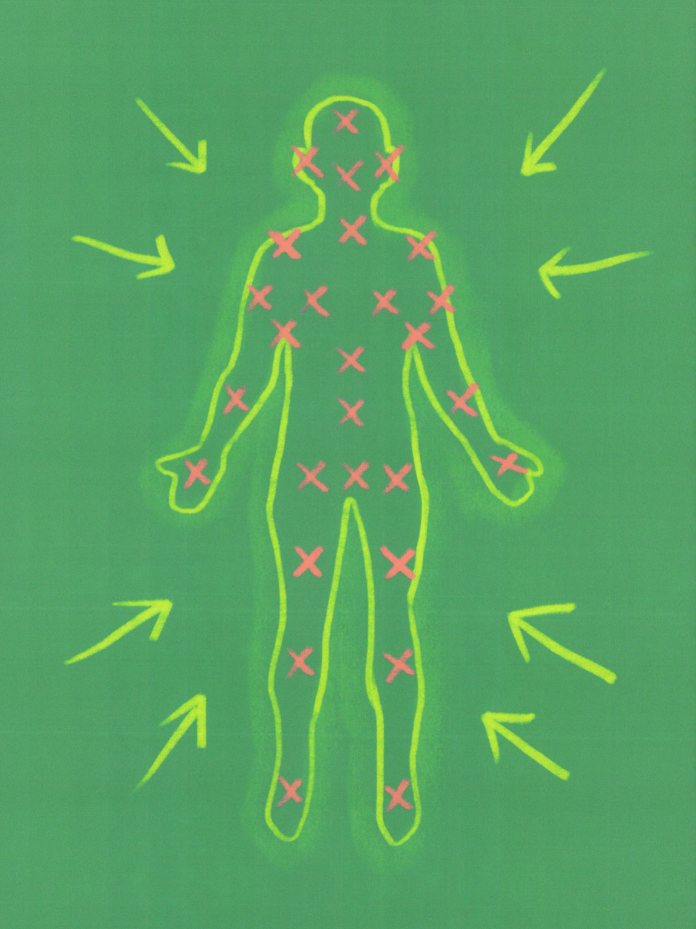

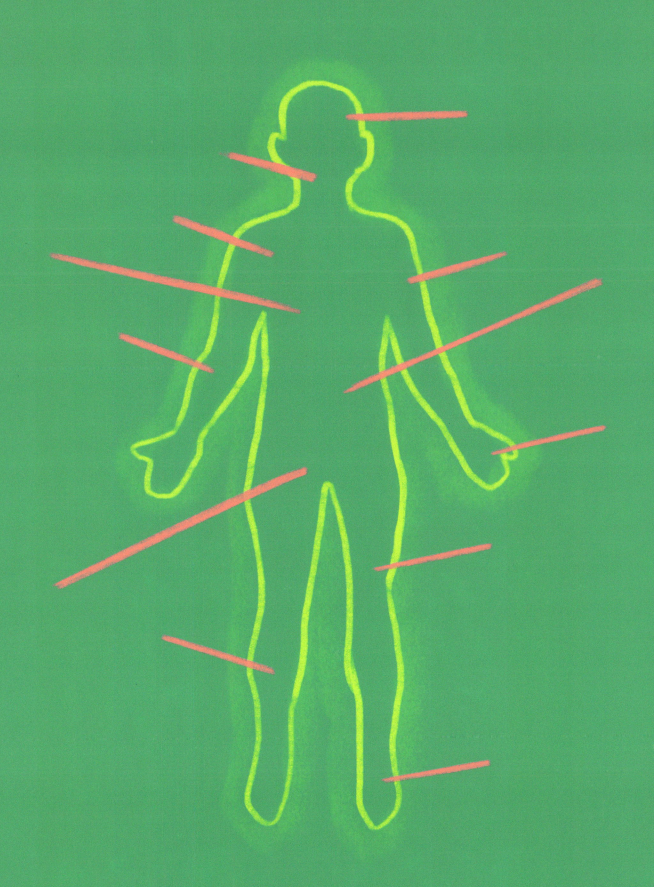

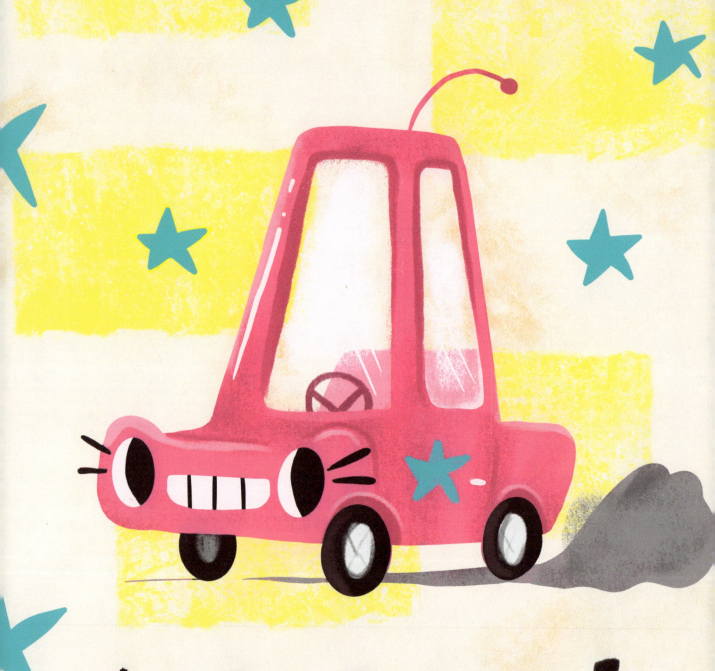

Did someone say QUICKLY?

BEEP! BEEP! Hi! I'm Addie the caddy, and I can show you how to alert someone if they touch your personal property!

First, scream, "NO!" and yell at the top of your lungs. Yelling will scare them, and it will also allow someone to help you.

On the count of three, yell out "No!" with me!
One...two...three..."NO!"

Great job!

Do you remember which parts of your body our friend Tai the Teddy told us that someone else needs your permission to touch? Can you show me by pointing at them in the picture?

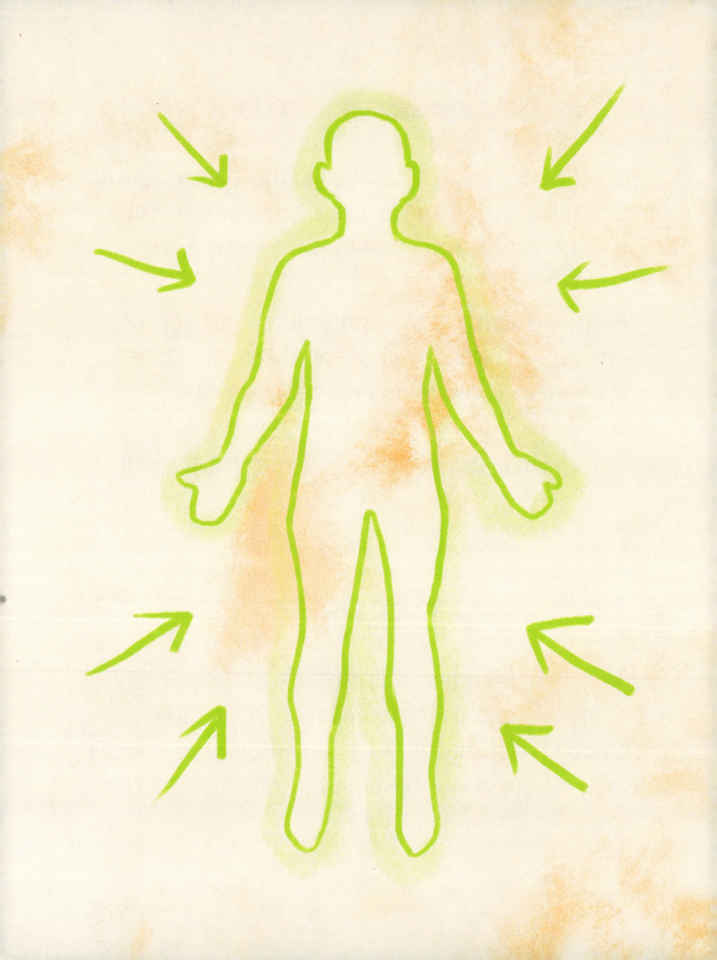

WOW! You remembered all of that? I'm sooo proud of you!

I want to tell you a secret—would you like to know it?

Awesome! The secret is...I think you're a star, just like me!

You should also know that secrets are not always good. Sometimes, people tell us BAD secrets that we should NOT keep to ourselves.

If someone touches any part of your body and asks you to keep it a secret, this is a BAD secret!

What should we do with bad secrets?

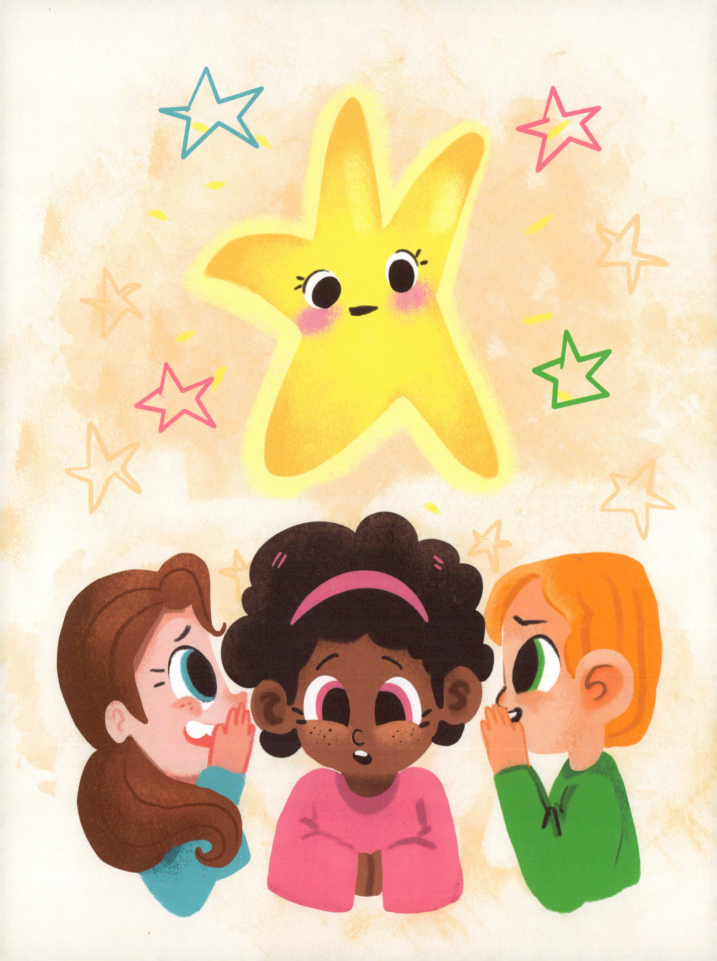

We have to tell our parents or another adult about the bad secret. Bad secrets can lead to bad things. Your parents will not be mad if you tell them about the bad secret.

If you are scared to tell your parents the secret, you and your mom, dad, or another adult can discuss what we call a code word!

A code word is a word we use to alert someone about an issue that's important to us.

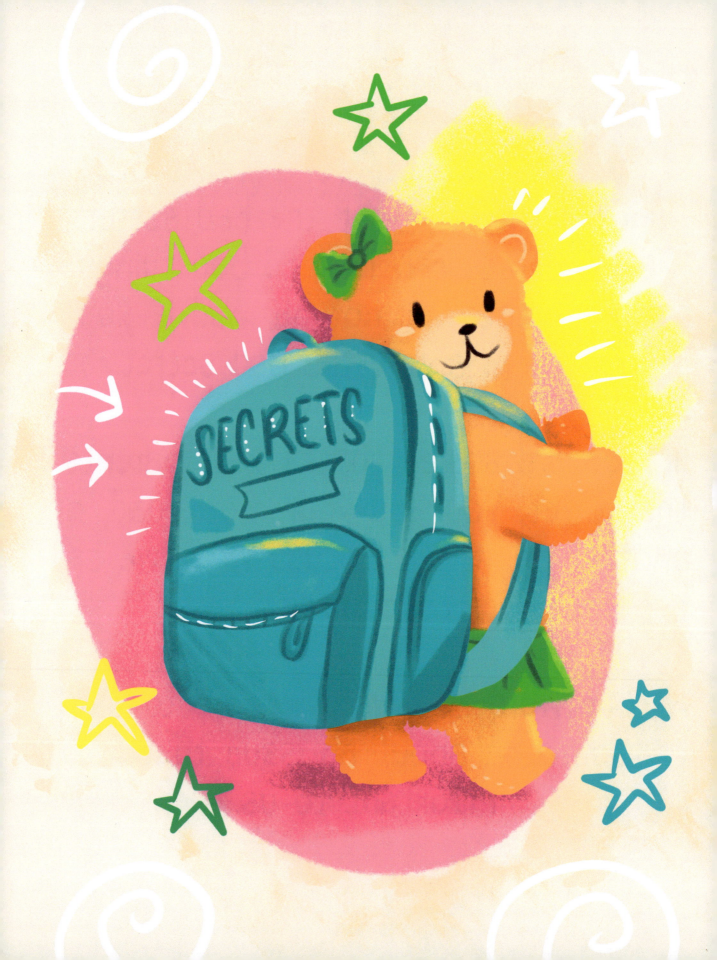

Let's drive the caddy down this road of code words. You and the adult you trust can pick one.

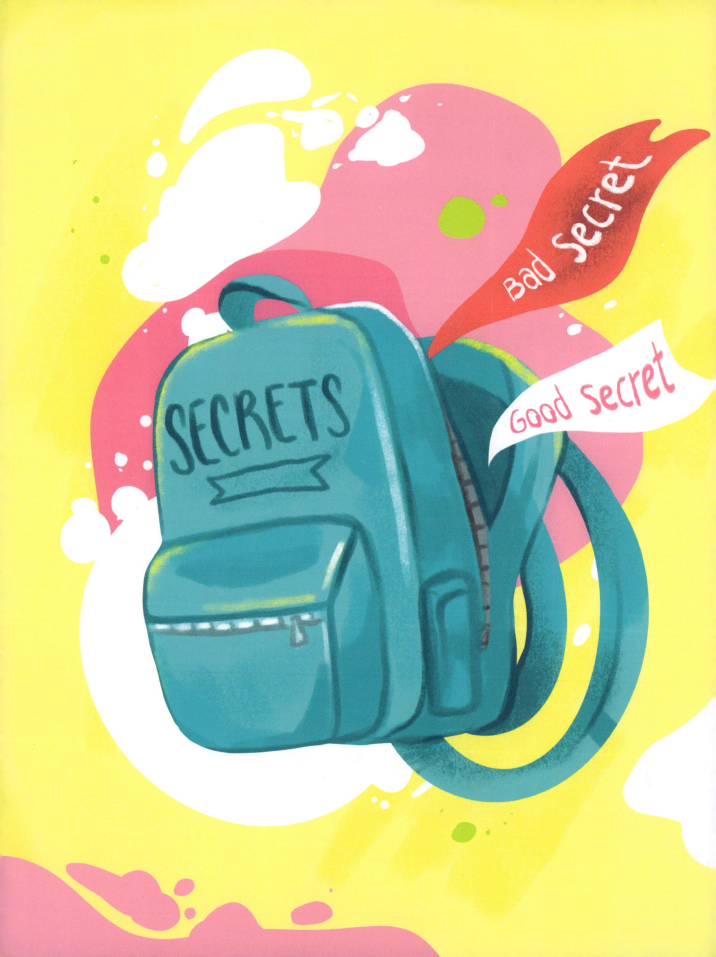

Bad Secret

Good Secret

Bad Secret

Good Secret

"I WISH I WAS A STARLIGHT"

"MY FOOT IS SORE"

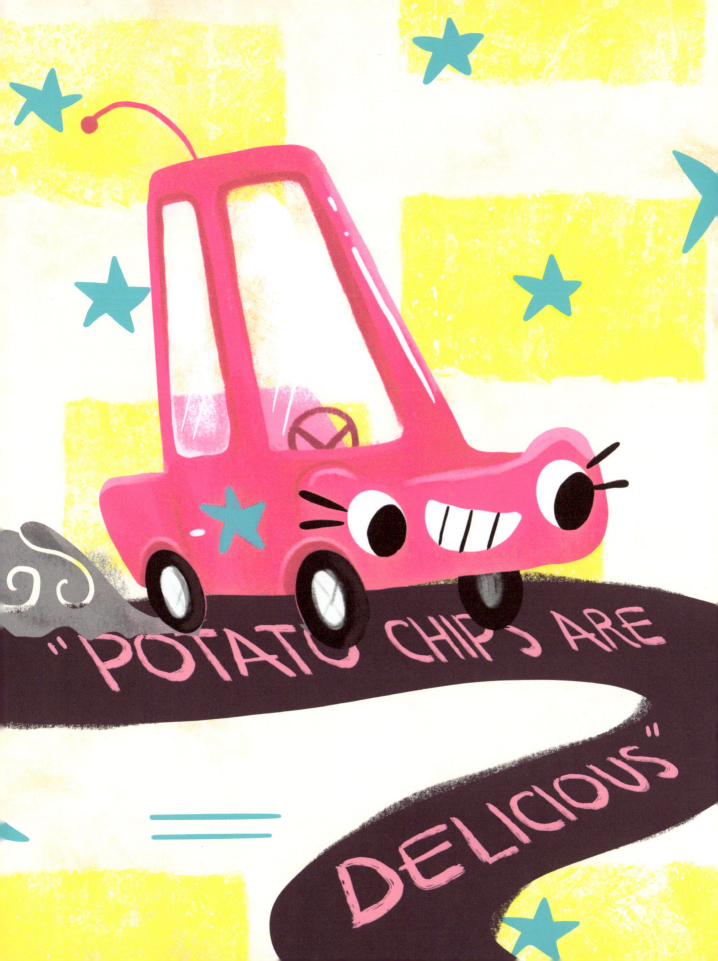

Now remember, we do NOT tell everyone the code word. The code word is for emergencies only. Do you know what the word "emergency" means?

The word emergency means a SERIOUS, unexpected, and often dangerous situation that requires IMMEDIATE action.

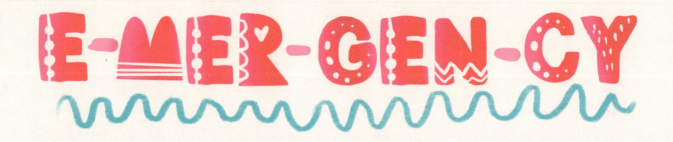

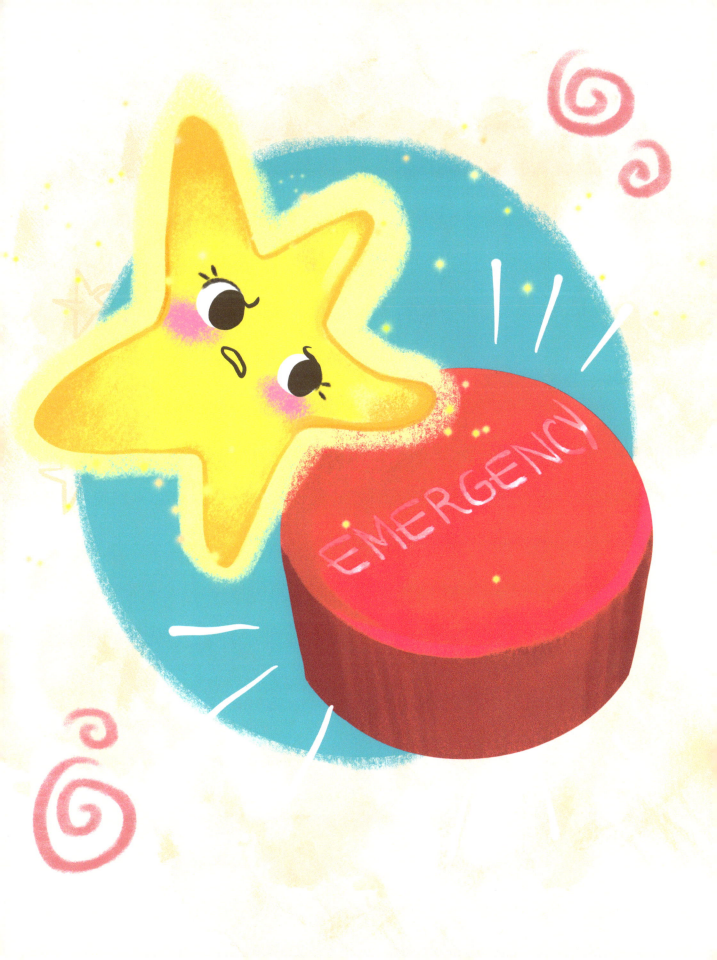

wow, you guys did so well! I'm so proud to call you my friends. After learning so much, how about we take a big picture!

Sayyyy cheeeeeeese.

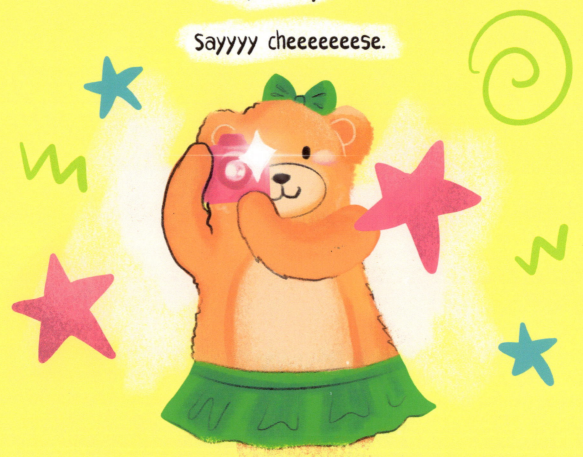

Pictures with our friends are great, but it's also important to remember that nobody should take a picture of us with no clothes on or touch our personal property.

It's also important to remember not to take pictures of anybody else without any clothes on or touch their personal property, either.

So, let's remember: NO to pictures, and nooo to bad secrets

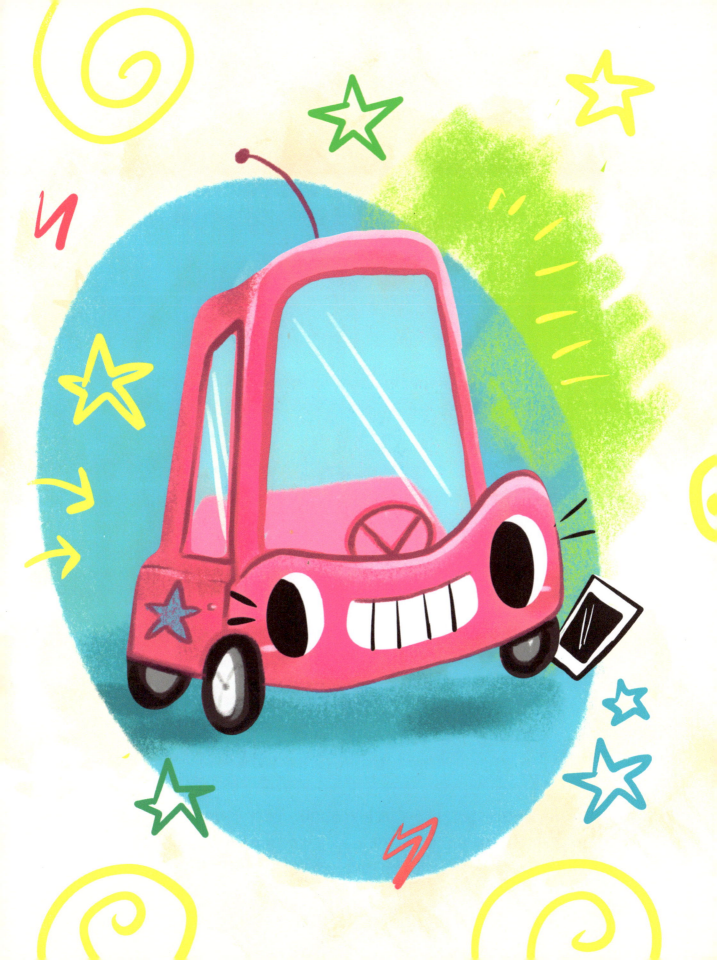

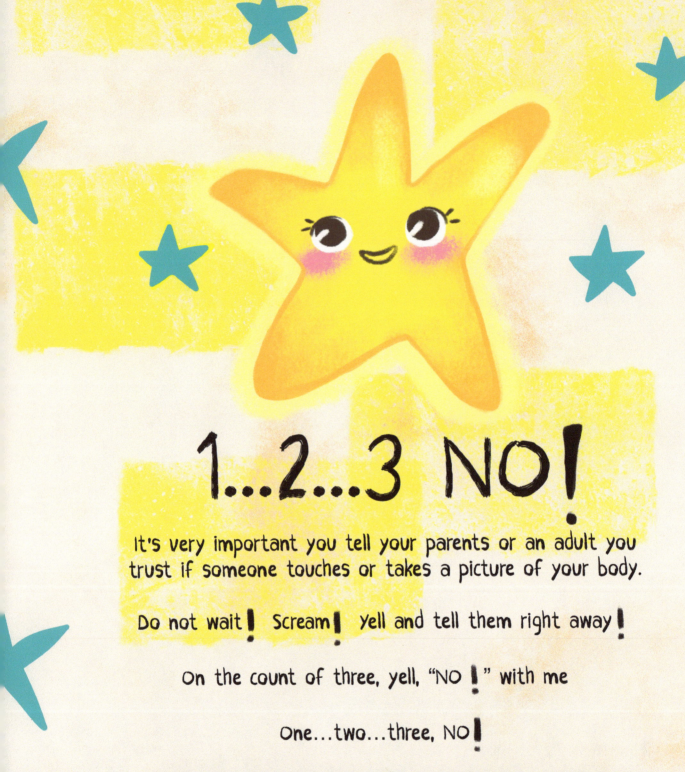

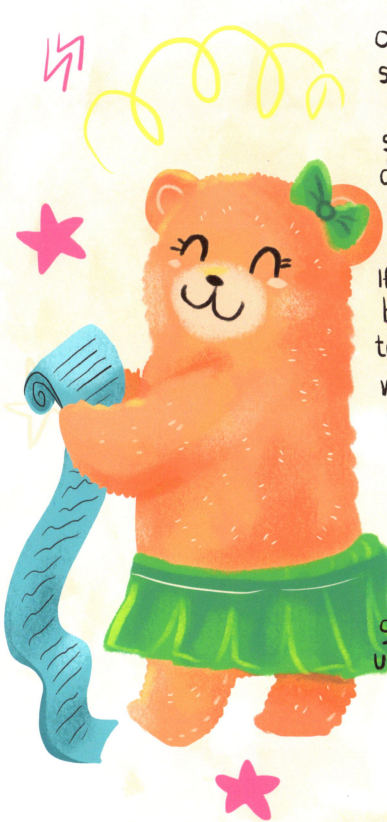

Our parents love us, so they will keep us safe. However, sometimes, parents do not believe their children.

If our parents don't believe us, we have to tell another adult we trust—someone who makes us feel safe.

Here's a list of people I trust: teachers, grandparents, aunts, uncles, police, nurses, and doctors. Can you tell me some people you trust?

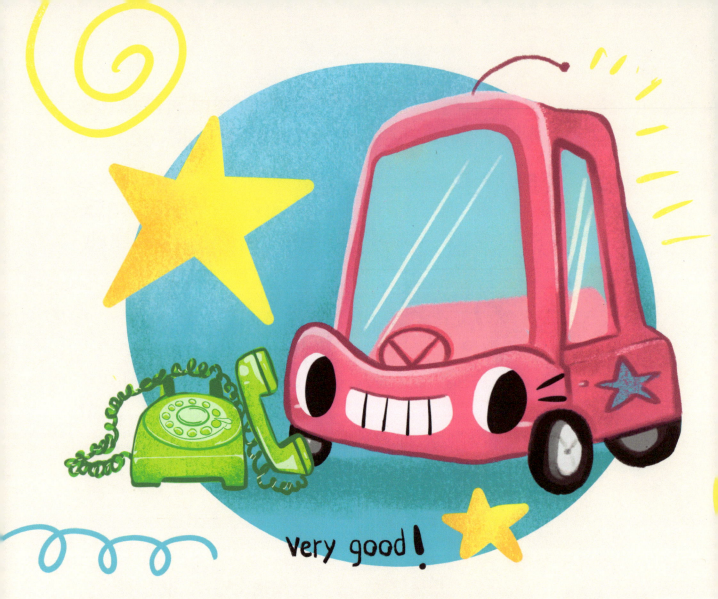

very good!

That's a great list of people you trust, and I am so happy for you! To be sure you can contact them if you need to, how about we write their phone numbers down, so we always have them? I've included very important numbers, too.

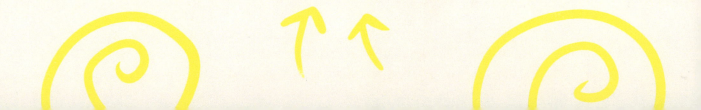

# Important numbers:

9-1-1 - Universal Emergency Number

800-422-4453 - Child Abuse Crisis Hotline Number

866-367-5544 - Child Sexual Abuse Crisis Hotline

1-800-799-SAFE (7233) - Domestic Violence Hotline

_____

_____

_____

Boys and girls, learning and talking with you has been absolutely amazing. We are so happy you allowed us to share some important information. But before we go, we need to repeat this information one more time to make sure you truly understand!

Remember,

1. Your body belongs to you; it is your personal property. Take a moment to name your body parts.
2. Absolutely NOBODY should touch your personal property without YOUR permission.
3. If anyone tries to touch you, yell NO very loudly, and tell someone — QUICKLY!
4. If someone tells you a BAD secret, tell your parents or an adult you trust.
5. Using a code word can help you tell your parents or trusted adults the bad secret: Do you remember your code word? Don't forget — we do NOT tell everyone our code word.
6. If someone tries to take a picture of your body, yell, "NO!"
7. You should never take a picture of someone else's body or TOUCH their body without their permission.
8. Tell your parents or a trusted adult if someone does any of these things we have talked about. Tell them QUICKLY.
9. If your parents or a trusted adult doesn't believe you, you need to find another trusted adult or choose a number from your list to call.
10. No means no!

...and you are a shining star!

CPSIA information can be obtained
at www.ICGtesting.com
Printed in the USA
BVHW021148210521
607870BV00005B/10